Hair Survival Guide 101:

A wondrous collection of hair care essays from real life experiences

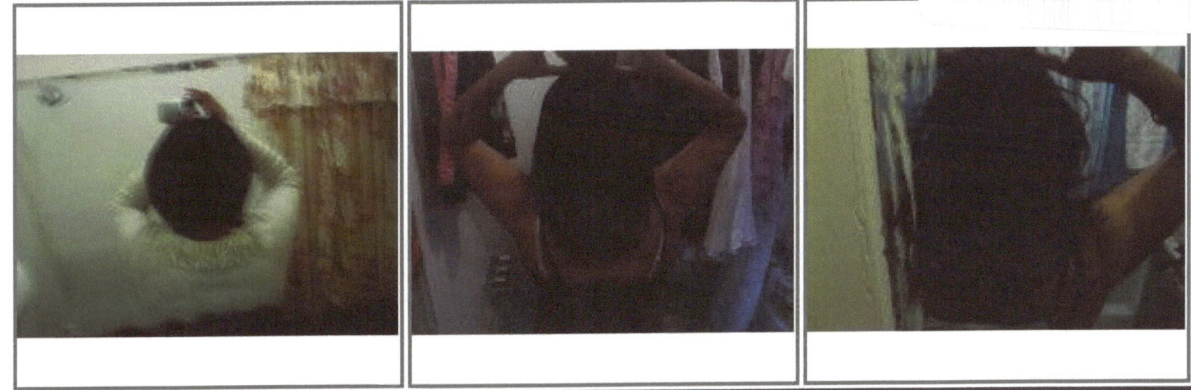

Continous hair growth from NL and beyond

By

Carmen S. Gonzalez, MS.Ed.

This book is dedicated to all of my hair sistas. Thanks for your continuous support. Without your help, I may have never acquired my new love for healthy hair and hair growth.

To my first hair teacher: My mom.

To my dad who pushed for me to not rely on extensions.

To my little sister who is one of my hair inspirations.

To my best friend, my fiancé for believing in all of my goals, including my hair goals.

It Starts with Pre-poo

Caring for the hair starts with the beginning of the process. A pre-poo a day keeps the scissor happy stylist away. The pre-poo is the barrier that stops the shampoo from stripping the hair. Pre-pooing is done on dry hair. This means that you are applying conditioner without any water.

Pre-poo can be concocted however you desire. Pre-poo can be done with a conditioner or an oil. It can also be made with both. Some use their favorite "cheepie" conditioners and mix it with their favorite oil. When you are lacking funds it is alright to use a conditioner from the dollar store.

Pre-pooing is not a long and extraneous process. Begin the pre-poo process by mixing your pre-poo in a large bowl or an old conditioner bottle. I prefer to mix it with coconut oil, almond oil, and cinnamon oil. Apply the pre-poo to your hair with your hands. Take each section of your hair and apply it section by section as if you were applying a chemical relaxer. Finally place a plastic cap or a hot towel on your hair. You may leave it on your hair all day if you please, but no shorter than 30 minutes for best results.

Pre-pooing is derived from the term shampooing. This process is done before the shampoo process. When in doubt remember that pre-pooing can be done to your liking. Some pre-poo by adding honey, but conditioner and oil has worked tremendously for my hair.

Pre-pooing the hair is the most important process of hair care. Pre-pooing is the part of the hair process that stops your hair from being stripped of its natural oils. Shampooing has been known to strip hair by making it very dry. Pre-pooing the hair protects it from the dryness caused by shampooing.

Shampooing is not what you may think it is…

After pre-pooing, the next stage of the hair care process is shampooing. Many feel that clean hair is extra suds. Have you ever been to the laundry mat and noticed the sign do not over sud the machine? Many think that over-sudding means that it is extra clean. Over sudding is applying a lot of soap.

When you wash your hair, remove the pre-poo by first applying a lot of water. Make sure that your hair is thoroughly cleansed by using water first. Make sure that your hair is wet from roots to ends. You should wet your hair for about three to four minutes. This is to ensure that your hair is completely wet and not just lightly moist in some sections.

Next, apply a quarter sized amount of shampoo to your hand and then the hair roots only. If your hair is less than shoulder length then apply about a dime sized amount of shampoo to your hand and then the hair roots. Do not rub vigorously. Be gentle with your hair and it will be kind to you.

After you shampoo your hair, it is important to not wash your hair for anything more than 1 more round. Some people feel that washing your hair more than 2 times makes it clean. Washing your hair more than 2 times removes the hair oils. You'd be surprised with how clean your hair can be with just two shampooing rounds. More shampoo does not make it clean. Do not use anything more than 2 rounds of shampoo. Do not use any more than 1 kind of shampoo on your hair at a time. You only need one shampoo.

Finally when shampooing, remember to rinse all of the shampoo out of your hair. Massage the roots as your remove the shampoo. You will notice that although you did not scrub the ends that the shampoo dripped down to the ends. Gently rinse the shampoo from your hair, root to end. Rinse your hair for about 4-5 minutes. This ensures that the hair is shampoo free.

In essence, there is misconception of what clean hair is. Clean hair is not over-cleansing with shampoo. It is also not washing the strands. The scalp is the real area that requires most of the cleansing; however, you are still cleaning the hair because the shampoo drips to the ends any way.

Conditioner is done with every wash...

Conditioner is done with every wash. Regardless of what many people believe, the conditioner is very important. Think of the conditioner as the fabric softener you put in your clothes. Conditioner is the part of the hair that not just leaves your hair soft and manageable, but also repairs possible damages from the environment and the shampoo.

Conditioning is done by applying it to wet hair. It is important to wet the hair for at least 3-4 minutes. If you rinsed your hair properly after shampooing your hair, then this part should be easy. I am asking you to wet your hair to make sure that you are not applying conditioner to shampoo.

Next, blot out a little of the water from the hair, but do not wring your hair like a rag. Your hair is not a rag. Blot your hair lightly and gently. This is so that when you apply the conditioner, the hair is conditioned and not the water.

Apply a quarter sized amount of conditioner to your hair from root to end. Massage the scalp as you are conditioning your hair. Do this for about 5 minutes. Conditioning the hair acts as a stimulating factor for hair growth. Conditioning can be done with any type of conditioner that you can afford and depending on your hair type. People with dry hair can benefit from a moisturizing conditioner. People with hair that is limp or fine can use more protein conditioner.

Finally conditioned hair does not stop here. Apply a deep conditioner section by section to the entire hair. Part each area and apply from root to end. Place a conditioning cap on the hair. Let it stay on your hair for about 15-30 minutes. You will love the texture of your hair after the conditioning process is complete. Your deep conditioner does not have to cost an arm and a leg. Deeping on your hair type, you may choose a moisturizing conditioner or a protein based conditioner. Regardless of the conditioner that you use, always finish by blotting the hair each time before applying the conditioner. The last conditioner that you should finish with is a leave- in conditioner.

In summary, regardless of the condition or type of hair, conditioner is important because it leaves the hair manageable. For those who want to maximize their hair growth, conditioning the hair is important. The reason is because conditioner keeps your hair protected from pollutants and other the harshness of chemicals from the environment.

Drying the hair

Whether you are air drying your hair in the summer or using a hand held or even a hooded dryer there are some do's and don'ts to drying the hair. Some people feel that air drying is the best thing that one can do for the hair. Some people feel that it leaves the hair crunchy so they turn to hand held or hooded dryers. The problem comes from over doing certain processes.

Before drying the hair regardless of what method you use, it is very important to apply some type of barrier to the hair. Using a leave-in that is specifically for hair before blowing or heating appliances is the best product to use. If you treat your hair well, it will be good to you. You may think that your hair does not need a protective barrier, but your hair will more than likely shed and fall excessively if you do not use some type of serum or cream that is meant for hair that is going to be blow dried or applied heat with. If you are hair drying your hair, applying a serum helps your hair dry frizz free. You may use a product that is specifically to minimize frizz.

Over using the hand held dryer is using direct heat. Direct heat is not the best heat that should be used for the hair. If you want to use some type of heat then you should be patient and use the roller set method depending on the length of the hair and sit under the dryer until the hair is completely dry. When using a hooded dryer, it is important to use the dryer on the medium setting. Using it on the highest setting is like cooking your hair. You will see crispy ends as the years progress with repeated exposure to direct or high heat. If you need to use direct heat then use the medium not the high setting. However, I do not recommend direct heat.

Air drying can be the best method to use if you live in a warmer climate or if it is warm outside. Air drying with rollers can be very beneficial. Air drying can keep the hair healthy, but for those on the go you must budget your time appropriately. Air drying the hair is drying the hair naturally without any heating agents: no heated dryer.

In short, drying the hair can be done with air drying, hooded dryer, or hand held dryer. Direct heat is not the best type of heat if you do not use it properly. Regardless of the method that you use to dry the hair, you must always use some type of protective agent. It can be a serum or any type of leave in that is made to protect the hair from the process of heat.

Air-dried hair

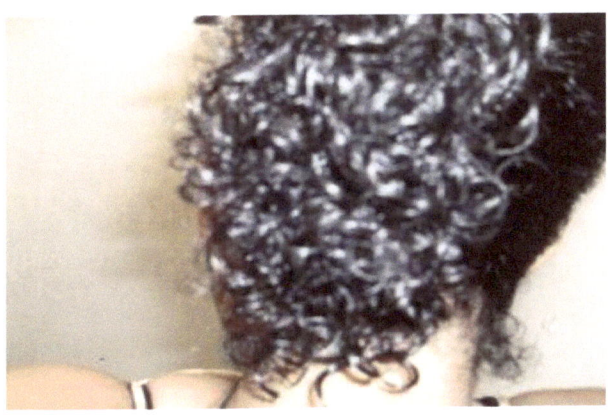

This style is achieved by using conditioner only wash method. No mousse or gel applied. Hair was dried naturally. No heat.

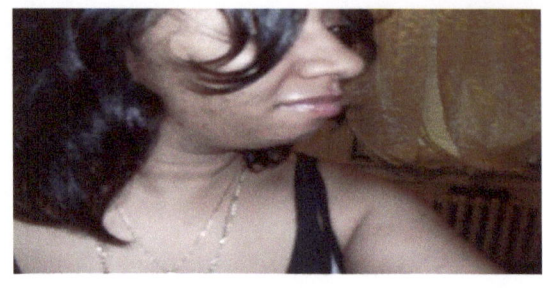Roller set only with no hand held blow-dryer. Hooded dryer used only

Protective Styling is Inevitable

There are many people who believe in letting the hair swing. Besides it looks pretty right. However, for many people letting the hair swing does not allow the hair to grow and prosper. Protective Styling is the secret to great lengths. I am not saying that protective styling should be done in silos, but it should be done. When done appropriately it can maximize hair growth potential.

First, protective styling is the act of hiding the ends to keep in moisture. For protective styling to work, it is very important to moisturize the hair with a moisturizing hair cream and sealing the ends with oil. You preferred moisturizer and oil is your choice. Be sure to use one that is for your hair type. Do not put more than a dime sized amount in your hair. Some products even remind you that you should put no more than a dime sized amount.

Some protective styles that I like to use are hair buns, and loose French braids. Any style that does not cause tension on the hair roots is alright. The idea is to not expose the ends of the hair while retaining the moisture.

Next, it is important to be consistent with protective styling. By staying consistent with anything especially protective styling you will see the difference and see that it really works for your hair. Some people even like to take pictures of their progress and keep a hair journal.

Some Protective Styles:

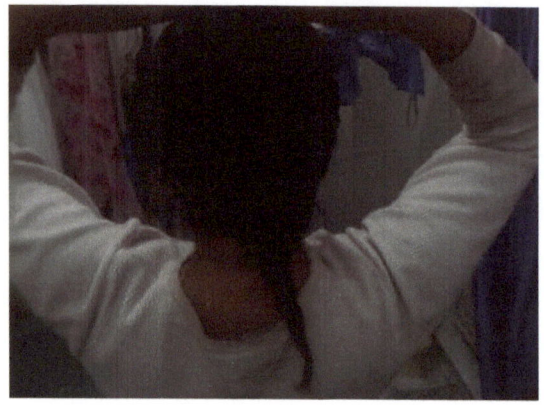 French braid. You can tuck in the

braid or leave it out.

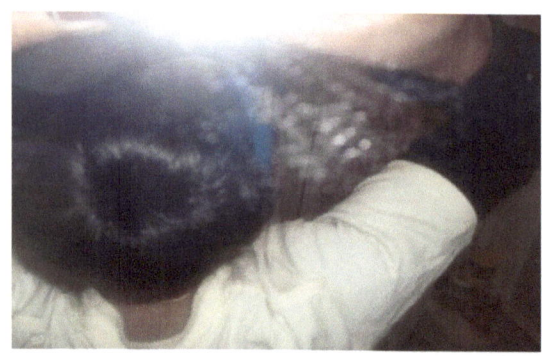 Ballet bun can be done with a

scrunchie on the bottom to cheat the thickness of the bun or without the

scrunchie. Scrunchie can be the color of your hair.

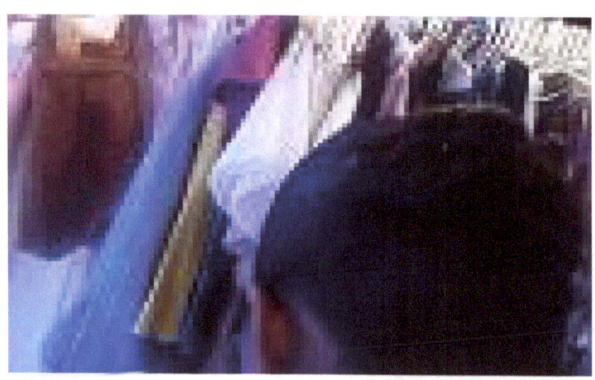

Bun done as a braid first then pinned down.

If you noticed, protective styling does not have to cost a lot of money. You do not have to go to a professional hair braider. You are your best beautician, because you know what kind of tension your hair needs. Protective Styling helps when you are gentle with your hair. None of these styles should hurt you. You can even go for chop sticks or other hair clips. Just as long as you do not use metal barrettes your hair will prosper. Metal Clips and barrettes hurt you and your hair because hair growth can be minimized due to breakage.

Moisturizing and Sealing should be done every day…

Moisturizer and oil should be applied to the hair every day. Moisturizing and oiling of the hair can be done to promote hair growth. Moisturizer should be applied mainly to the ends, but can be done from root to end. Oil should be applied to the ends only. This is the process of oiling and sealing.

This is easier said than done. Moisturizing and oil should be practiced daily to minimize breakage. Moisturizing should not be done every second of the day. It should, however, be done at least one to two times a day. The reason is because more than likely you will leave home at least twice. When you leave home and then come back, more than likely you are exposing your hair to harsh air and it can dry it out. When you get ready for bed you should always apply oil.

Think of moisturizing and oiling of the hair has any part of the body. When you do not lubricate your skin, it becomes dry. When it dries out it becomes scaly and ashy. Your hair will fall out over time if it is not moisturized, especially if it is afro textured. Relaxed hair especially needs moisture and oil applied to it, since chemical relaxers can dry the hair.

Finally, if your hair is extremely dry, you can fix this problem by doing a process called the baggy method. The baggy method is done by creating a pony tail. Then, attach a sandwich baggy or a clear conditioning cap to the ends only.

In essence, by combining the baggy method with moisture and oil, you are on your way to well moisturized and oiled hair. By doing this consistently, you will notice that your hair will be more manageable and less dry. Your choice of moisturizer and conditioner can be based on your own preference and what works best for your hair.

Wrapping the Hair

Wrapping the hair is very critical. When wrapping the hair it is very important to tie the hair down with a bobby pin on each side if it is relaxed. Wrapping the hair done is also called the doobie on some parts of the world. The wrapping affect is created by wrapping the hair around the entire head. The wrap helps because it creates a natural bump on the end. After the wrap is done, by using a comb and a large wig brush, then tie the hair down with a silk and satin scarf and two bobby pins: one on each end.

Wrapping the hair at night make the hair not only look appealing when you wake up, but it helps you keep your hair on your head if you suffer from excessive dryness. After you moisturize your hair before bed time, then the final step before bed time is the wrap and the scarf method.

Wrapping the hair at night is the method of choice when you do not want a lot of tension on the hair root. Wrapping the hair at night does not hurt you hair. If you are a wild sleeper then try keeping the hair over your eye brows at night when you are tying the scarf on your head. Continue to clip each end down at night.

The large wig brush can work like a charm along with a wide took comb when you are wrapping your hair around your head at night. I prefer to wrap my hair with this type of brush and comb over the boar bristle brush or small tooth comb because there is less tension on my hair. It is important, however, not to overdue the brushing and the combing. Get the hair straight the first time and then leave it alone. Less is better when it comes to brushing and combing.

In short, by keeping the hair wrapped at night, you will watch your hair prosper because you were able to keep your hair on your head. By keeping the scarf on your hair at night you are minimizing the friction on your hair against your pillowcase. The less friction, the better your hair will be. Continue to wrap your hair and night after moisturizing and sealing and you will see the benefits of these combined methods.

Trims and Scissor Happy Stylist

If a stylist does not respect your hair then they do not respect you. When you go to a stylist and you want a trim, try using the term dust the ends. A dust is exactly what it says a dust. Think of granules of dust that are collected on furniture after a set amount of time. Dusting should not cause you to go from Shoulder length (SL) back to Neck Length (NL) in the matter of seconds. When this happens you were disrespected.

Anyone can grow hair to any length that they wish. Do not let someone tell you, your ends are dry I am trimming your ends. You may just need conditioner. Conditioner is usually the answer in my case. Trims just help the hair keep a style. Trims do not grow the hair. If it is meant to grow the hair then it would not get shorter with every cut.

Scissor happy stylists get more money for a cut. If you want to grow your hair out a specific way then you can trim to your liking but it is not necessary. I can remember all of my progress getting cut. I got layers and I did not want them. This taught me that sometimes stylists just do not care. So I began caring for my own hair.

I went from this… Neck Length in 2008

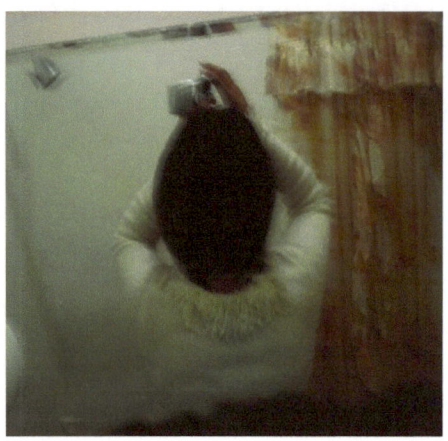

To Arm pit length by the end of 2010/ beginning of 2011

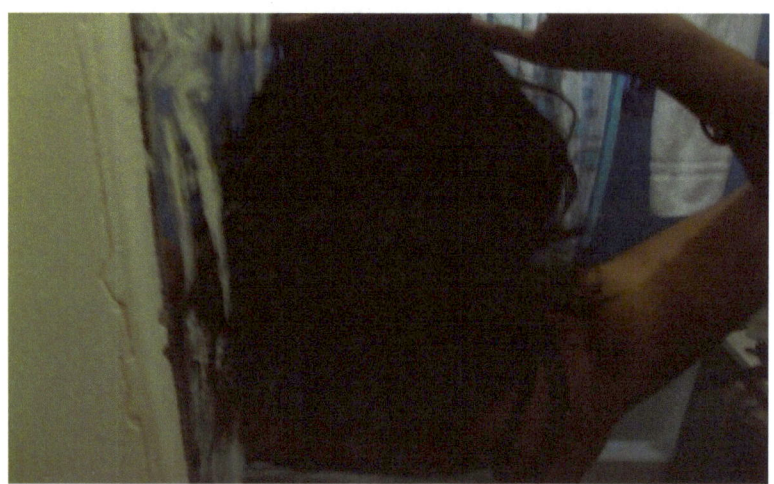

This was created by taking a stand with my hair and not letting anyone control what I wanted. You have to know what you want. I want growth and cutting will not help my hair.

In essence, trimming the hair is not cutting progress. If you tell your beautician you want your ends dusted then it is a dust not a cut. If they cut then they do not respect you. Keep looking for a new one. Try a long hair specialist. If you do not have any luck, then try trimming your own ends or finding someone else that you trust. It can even be a family member or another loved one.

Moisture Protein Balance is inevitable…

Everyone needs some type of protein and moisture. The question is how much how much do we need in our hair. Some say listen to your hair. They are correct. If your hair is dry and kind of brittle then you may need moisturizing shampoo and moisturizing conditioner. If your hair is limp and kind of life less then you may need protein shampoo and conditioner.

If you do not know the difference, every newbie to the hair care game tries to alternate between moisture and protein. Learn what your hair likes and does not like. If you like how your hair feels then your hair will benefit from either more moisture or more protein. Take notes in a journal. How does it look and feel.

If it is shedding a little you may need garlic shampoo and conditioner. The important part in this matter is to follow up with moisturizing deep conditioner. No one will know your hair better than you know your hair.

Regardless of what your hair is doing you need to balance both protein and moisture. After a chemical relaxer, your hair will need some type of protein about 3 weeks later. After about 6 weeks your hair may begin to revert. You may benefit from a different type of protein called keratin.

In essence, listening to your hair needs is the most important part of hair care. Whether your hair is shedding, dry, limp, or lifeless, you can always find a remedy for your hair at home. By listening to your hair, you will minimize the amount of visits to the salon and save on hair trims and cuts. You will realize that all you needed was a simple change in conditioner and shampoo.

www.ingramcontent.com/pod-product-compliance
Lightning Source LLC
Chambersburg PA
CBHW041531280526
45792CB00004B/1460